Steps4Health Grill and Garden
20 Tweets
to a Healthy Tailgate

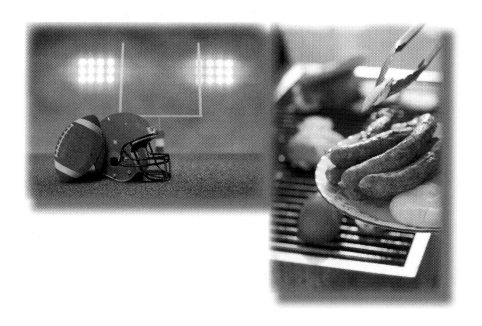

Presented by B. Ann Matthews

authorHOUSE®

AuthorHouse™ LLC
1663 Liberty Drive
Bloomington, IN 47403
www.authorhouse.com
Phone: 1-800-839-8640

Published by AuthorHouse 04/11/2014

ISBN: 978-1-4918-6247-6 (sc)
ISBN: 978-1-4918-6250-6 (e)

Library of Congress Control Number: 2014902388

DEDICATION

To football fans and grill masters,
who celebrate the game of football!

This book is also dedicated to my family
and friends
who enjoy their food, hot off the grill!

INTRODUCTION

Are you a football fan? Are you a grill master? Live for going to the game on the weekends? Can't wait to see the crew for NFL Sundays?

Steps4Health Grill and Garden, 20 Tweets to a Healthy Tailgate encourages healthy eating at the pre-game party! Whether or not you tailgate at the stadium or grill at home, you will find this book informative and humorous!

This playbook contains motivation to KICK START your new diet, exercise goals or maintain your current healthy lifestyle, while enjoying the football game!

LIVE LAUGH LOVE LEARN

GAME DAY!

Rise Up!

Soar! Score!

Activate your playbook!

Elevate your game-

You can reach your diet and #fitness goals!

Rise Up!

Soar! Score!

Accelerate, drive yourself-

To reach your nutrition diet, and #fitness goals!

Rise Up!

Accelerate, Drive, Run the ball-

Let healthy #food be your fuel injection!

BREAKFAST FOR CHAMPIONS

Do you serve a #breakfast for champions?

How do you start your morning?

What's in your bowl for breakfast?

Do you like oatmeal or grits in your bowl?

What do you add to your breakfast bowl?

Do you add fresh blueberries, bananas, or walnuts?

What's in your bowl at your college #gameday party?

A bowl of crudities, low fat chips or pita breads-

A bowl of #salad—Caesar, chief, mixed green salad?

A bowl of salsa, hummus, artichoke, or spinach cheese dips?

You be the referee!

Here is the play—TACOS!

How do you call it?—How do you like your tacos?

With chicken, beef, fish, or beans?

Hard shell or soft shell—

With lettuce or shredded cabbage-

With onions, peppers, guacamole or sour cream?

Hot Potato, Hot Potato, Pass the #ball-

How do you grill potatoes?

Hot Potato, Hot Potato,

Pass the hot potato, Pass the ball!

GARDEN

The start of planting season for some-

Do you have a green thumb?

Pardon the pollen . . .

Remove the leaves that have fallen-

And start your #garden!

Mary, Mary, Quite Contrary

How does your #garden grow?

Create a veggie delight-

Plant some seeds, pull the weeds,

Water, Sun, almost done,

With a row of bell peppers,

A row of green beans,

And the largest, brightest red tomatoes,

You have ever seen!

Mary, Mary, Quite Contrary

How does your garden grow?

Do you know,

How to sow, a salsa garden?

Bend your knees, throw some seeds,

Water, sun, almost done,

Then comes peppers, tomatoes, onions, and cilantro!

The season has changed-

Fall is upon us, so are the leaves,

What are your favorite leafy greens?

How do you like your greens?

In a #salad or sautéed?

Kale or collards?

Did you have your leafy greens today?

Swish Healthy Greens

Swish them in water!

Swish them in a pan!

Swish them in a smoothie!

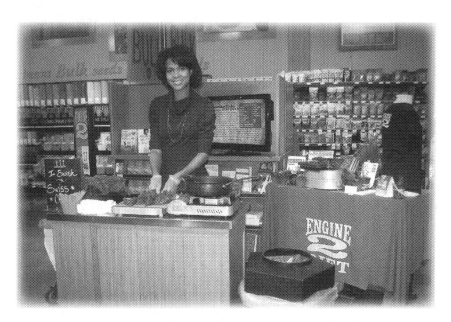

SWISH Presentation

GRILL

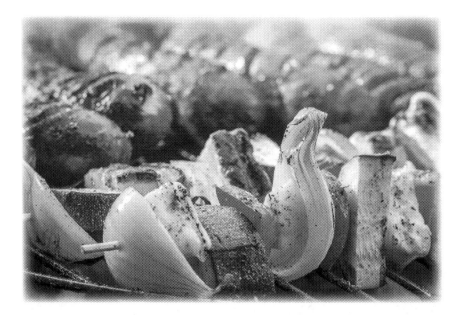

First Down

Tailgating?

Watching the big #game?

Make a first down by decreasing your fat intake!

"Trim the fat" from your diet—

Substitute non-fat or low fat items for high fat items!

Who is going to the Super Bowl!?

Who will be the Super Bowl challengers?

What are your #food, diet challenges?

Reduce sugar intake?

Increase fresh #fruit and salads?

You can OVERCOME your food challenges!

Planning your first tailgate or pre-game party?

Game Day Menu Ideas

Starters

Grapes, chilled

Corn chips, low-fat, low sodium

Celery sticks, carrots

Dip: ranch dressing, salsa, or blue cheese

Salad

Fruit salad

Green salad

Sides

Corn on cob, grilled

Potato, grilled

Vegetable kebabs grilled

Main Dish

Grilled BBQ chicken breast, leg quarters

Hamburgers, Steak, Chops

Sausages, Hot Dogs

Salmon, Tuna steak, Halibut

Dessert

Pineapple slices, grilled

Beverages

Water, lemonade, beer*

When consuming alcohol, drink responsibility, don't drink and drive!

STEPS4HEALTH FAVORITE GRILLED RECIPES

Seasoned Butter

For grilled corn or potato

Add the following to 1 stick of unsalted, softened butter

- Minced garlic, chili powder, celery leaves, coriander, cumin, and minced red and yellow bell pepper

- Fold items into softened butter

- Roll seasoned butter into wax paper. Twist ends and chill in refrigerator.

Green Salad

Mix the following ingredients in a salad bowl!

- Mixed greens, Craisins, Mandarin Oranges, Walnuts, Vinaigrette Dressing

Black Bean Burgers

- Place a black bean (vegan) burger on a pre-oiled grill. Warm on both sides.

- Top with lettuce, salsa, and a bun!

Grilled Tuna Teriyaki

- Marinade Ahi Tuna steaks in teriyaki sauce or teriyaki ginger sauce for 30 minutes.

- Place marinated tuna steaks on pre-oiled grill.

- Splash fresh squeezed orange juice on tuna steaks 3 minutes before done.

- Season with salt and pepper!

Beef Fajitas

- Season grilled sirloin tip with Mc-Cormick's Fajita Seasoning Packet.

- Remove sirloin tip from grill when done.

- Let meat sit for five minutes.

- Slice grilled sirloin tip into strips.

- Place sirloin strips into warm tortillas with grilled onion and green bell pepper. Add sour cream and/or guacamole!

STEPS4HEALTH SUPER BOWL BLITZ

Football is about fitness and #teamwork and on Super Bowl Sunday,

The food is important too!

Get in the game with Steps4Health Grill and Garden-

Grilled #Salmon Recipe: Dijon mustard, lime juice, dill and parsley-

No matter where, nor how you enjoy the game, from paper #football,

To making plays from your playbook,

We love the big game of football!

Go Outside

Great day to be outside!

Start your engines!

#Water bottle READY,

Sunscreen SET,

Seatbelt GO!

SUN SMART SKIN HEALTH FROM DOWN UNDER

#Health experts from Australia tell us to:

Slip on a shirt,

Slop on #sunscreen,

Slap on a hat,

Seek shade or shelter,

Slide on some sunnies (sunglasses)!

Slip, Slop, Slap, Seek, Slide, if you are outside in the sun!

KNOW YOUR NUMBERS

Watching #sports today?

What is the score of the game?

Are you keeping score with your blood pressure?

Know your numbers!

The numbers 120/80 are the ones you should aim to keep your blood pressure,

Record your blood pressure numbers and share with your doctor!

Exercise, #diet, and lifestyle changes can control blood pressure.

SCREEN, SWEAT, AND SHINE!

Get screened today!

Screen—See your doctor for age appropriate tests!

Sweat—Stay physically active everyday!

Shine—Spread the word about your #health success!

Vow to maintain your good health,

And help others improve their health!

Screen, Sweat, Shine!

TAILGATING

Shuffle, Shuffle, Shift, Stir, Replace-

New grill? New Menu?

How do you keep your grill game fresh?

SEASONINGS AT THE TAILGATE

What do you use to season your #food @ your tailgate party?

Don't let too much salt keep you on the sidelines!

Some suggestions:

Garlic

Onion Powder

Red and Black Pepper

Hot Pepper Sauce

Fresh horseradish

Vinegar

Lemon or lime juice

National Institute of Health and the American Heart Association suggests using herbs and salt free spices and seasoning to reduce your sodium intake.

Simple and Easy Marinades for Grilling

* Lime juice and garlic for seafood

* Orange juice and teriyaki sauce for chicken or beef

* Italian dressing for vegetables

Be the CEO of your Diet!

Balance the amount of calories you eat with the amount of calories you burn!

Food Selection

When choosing food for your tailgate/pre-game party, choose nutritious foods!

THE ABC'S OF VITAMINS IN FOODS!

Vitamin A—Access to fresh orange vegetables is important!

Vitamin B—Let your diet be your multi-vitamin!

Vitamin C—See your way to a stronger Immune System!

Vitamin D—Choose a diet with dairy and foods high in nutrients!

Vitamin E—Expand your diet by adding nuts and seeds!

Do you exercise before work or school?

Haces ejercico antes de ir a la escuela o al trabajo?

What is your morning exercise routine?

Cual es tu retina de ejercico en las mananas?

If you go to the gym, walk outside, view a yoga DVD,

Don't forget your towel or water bottle.

Si vas a la gymnacio, caminas afuera, miras tus videoa de yoga,

No te olvides de tu toalla y tu botella de agua.

WALKING

Walk the dog-

Walk the campus-

Walk the track-

Add walking to your #fitness routine!

No matter what the weather is you can always—

Walk the mall!

STEPS4HEALTH THEME SONG

What #music is on your exercise playlist?

Steps4Health theme song is Step by Step by the late, great, Whitney Houston.

Add it to your #music playlist!!

REFRESH YOURSELF

Shape Up!—Refresh your #fitness routine!

Motivate!—Refresh your workout #music playlist!

Cleanse!—Refresh your digestive system!

Stretch!—Refresh your morning and afternoon jog!

Kids Corner
Children, Let's Move Song

Children, Let's Move!

Let's Move-

Let's Move-

Let's Move our bodies!

Use your feet to kick the ball-

Use your knees to skip hopscotch-

Use your arms to turn the rope-

Use your tummy to hula hoop-

Let's Move!

Let's Move!

Let's Move our bodies!

Use your back to jump up high-

Use your elbows to run, run fast-

Snap your fingers to keep the beat-

Wave your hands to dance silly, willy!

Let's Move!

Let's move our bodies!

OTHER #HEALTH TIPS

Handwashing-

How many times have you washed your hands today?

Keeping hands clean is one of the most important ways to prevent the spread of infection and illnesses.

Lavarse las manos

Cuantas veces te has lavado las manos hoy?

Mantener tus manos limpias es una de las maneras mas importantes para prevenir el contajio de infecciones y enfermedades

12 Steps to #Food Safety for your Football Pre-Game Party or Tailgate!

1. Keep raw meat separate from your breads, fruits, or vegetables. Place raw meat in a separate plastic bag.

2. Follow USDA Food Safety Guidelines: Clean, Separate, Cook, Chill!

   These next steps are if you are traveling to the big game and/or carrying food to another location . . .

3. Place food in a cooler, right from the refrigerator.

4. Chill food, at or below 40 degrees, in a cooler with ice/ice packs.

5. Have separate coolers for beverages and perishables and meat.

6. Keep cooler in shade, out of direct sunlight.

7. Bring clean water for food prep, and cleaning; pack wipes and hand sanitizer for cleaning surfaces and hands!

8. Avoid food poisoning! When food is finishing cooking on the grill, use clean utensils to remove from grill and place on clean plates. Boil liquid marinade first before placing it on cooked, prepared food.

9. Do not let food sit on counter or picnic area in 90 degree temps for more than one hour! Keep chilled!

10. Use a food thermometer to take the internal temp of the meat while it is on the grill!

Ground Beef	160° degrees
Poultry	165° degrees
Steaks	145° degrees
Pork, Lamb, Veal Chops	145° degrees

1. Wear sunscreen and a hat if you are outside grilling!

2. Remember the US Department of Food Safety tells us to Clean, Separate, Cook, Chill food for safety!

Call the Food Hotlines below if you have any questions:

USDA Meat and Poultry Hotline
1-888-674-6854

FDA Safe Food Hotline 1-888-723-3366

CDC Food Poisoning 1-800-232-4636

Or email a food safety expert with your questions at mphotline.fsis@usda.gov

Signs and Signals

Have you had much success with your diet and/or fitness plan?

What are some signs and signals of a successful diet and fitness plan?

- Weight loss?

- Normal blood glucose level?

- Increase physical activity level?

- Other positive changes?

Personal Note Section

Tailgate/Pre-Game Football Party Prep To Do List:

People to Invite/Invitation List:

Friends

Family

Co-Workers

Neighbors

Menu

Equipment

Grill

Food storage

Other

Personal Note Section

Your Favorite Team:

Team Colors:

Team Mascot:

Team Song/Chant:

YOUR DIET AND FITNESS GOALS

I want to reduce (sugar) (fat) (sodium) in my diet by substituting the following foods _____.

I want to add more physical activity to my weekly schedule by doing (activity) for (minutes).

I want to consume more fruits and veggies in my diet.

My current blood pressure level is:

My current blood glucose level is:

My next appointment with my health care provider is:

REFERENCES

- National Institutes of Health (NIH)

- American Heart Association (AHA)

- Mayo Clinic

- Centers for Disease Control and Prevention (CDC)

- United States Food and Drug Administration (USDA)

- UGA Extension

- National Football League (NFL)

- White House Task Force on Childhood Obesity; Let's Move Initiative